THE 48 LAWS OF POWER

ROBERT GREENE

(A CONCISE AND PRECISE SUMMARY)

Children's Guides

BY

Tomas Santiago

About Robert Greene

Robert Greene was born on May 14, 1959, in Los Angeles, California. His most famous compositions often center on themes of political or sexual intrigue. The 48 Laws of Power, The Art of Seduction, 33 Tactics for War, The 50th Law, and Mastery are only five of Greene's books that have become international bestsellers. His work has been featured in publications like Forbes, New York Times, CNN, New York Times Magazine, USA Today, Newsweek, Los Angeles Times, Huffington Post, Business Insider, Fast Company, Slate, Business Week, and XXL. Greene has made appearances on the Today Show, CNBC, ABC, and MTV News.

Copyright @2023 by Tomas Santiago- All Rights Reserved

This is NOT the official synopsis or analysis of the work in question. This summary and analysis was not written by the author or publisher of the book being discussed and should not be construed as such.

Both the publisher and the author of this book make no express or implied guarantees about the accuracy, completeness, or suitability of the material included within. Prices and details are subject to change at any time without notice.

With the exception of the limited circumstances described in Sections 107 and 108 of the United States Copyright Act of 1976, no part of this publication may be reproduced, stored in a retrieval system, or transmitted in any form or by any means, electronic, mechanical, photocopying, scanning, recording, or otherwise, without the express, written permission of the Publisher or Author.

CONTENTS

Introduction to The 48 Laws of Power 8

Law 1: 10

Do Not Outshine the Master 10

Law 2: 10

Be Wary of Friends and Learn to Use Your Enemies 10

Law 3: 11

Hide Your Intentions 11

Law 4: 11

Say Less Than Is Necessary 11

Law 5: 12

Guard Your Reputation with Your Life 12

Law 6: 13

Court Attention at all Cost 13

Law 7: 13

Have Others Do The Work, but Always Take the Credit 13

Law 8: 14

Make Others Come to You 14

Law 9: 15

Win Actions, Not Through Argument 15

Law 10: 16

Don't Be Infected by the Unhappy and Unlucky 16

Law 11: 17

Keep People Dependent on You 17

Law 12: 18

Use Selective Honesty and Generosity to Neutralize Your Enemies ... 18

Law 13: 18

Appeal to Other's Self-Interest, Not Their Mercy or Gratitude 18

Law 14: 19

Act Like a Friend, Work Like a Spy 19

Law 15: 19

Completely Crush Your Enemy 19

Law 16: 20

Absence Increases Respect and Honor 20

Law 17: 21

Be Occasionally Unpredictable to Keep Others in Suspended Terror . 21

Law 18: 22

Never Build Fortresses to Protect Yourself 22

Law 19: 23

Understand Who You're Dealing With, and Don't Offend the Wrong Person 23

Law 20: 24

Do Not Commit to Others 24

Law 21: 25

Play Dumber Than Your Mark 25

Law 22: 25

Use Surrender to Turn Weakness Into Power 25

Law 23: 26

Concentrate Your Forces 26

Law 24: 26

Play the Perfect Courtier 26

Law 25: 27

Re-Create Yourself 27

Law 26: 28

Keep Your Hands Clean 28

Law 27: 29

Take Advantage of People's Need to Believe 29

Law 28: 30

Act with Boldness, Not Timidity 30

Law 29: 31

Plan Until You Reach the End 31

Law 30: 32

Make your Accomplishments Seem Effortless 32

Law 31: 32

Make Others Play with the Cards You Deal 32

Law 32: 33

Play to Others' Fantasies 33

Law 33: 34

Discover Others' Weaknesses 34

Law 34: 35

If You Want to Be Treated Like a King, Act Like One 35

Law 35: 36

Master the Art of Timing 36

Law 36: 37

Ignoring What You Cannot Have Is the Best Revenge 37

Law 37: 38

Create Compelling Spectacles 38

Law 38: 38

Think Whatever You Want, But Behave Like Others 38

Law 39: 39

To Catch More Fish, Stir Up the Waters 39

Law 40: 39

Despise the Free Lunch 39

Law 41: 40

Avoid Stepping Into a Great Man's Shoes 40

Law 42: 40

Take Down the Shepherd and the Sheep Will Scatter 40

Law 43: 41

Work on the Hearts and Minds of Others 41

Law 44: 42

Use the Mirror Effect to Disarm 42

Law 45: 42

Preach the Need for Change, But Make Change Gradual 42

Law 46: 43

Do Not Appear to Be Too Perfect 43

Law 47: 43

In Victory, Learn When to Stop 43

Law 48: 44

Be Formless 44

INTRODUCTION TO THE 48 LAWS OF POWER

Robert Greene was a successful but unfulfilled Hollywood writer when he began tinkering with the ideas that would become The 48 Laws of Power. This allowed him to people-watch the rich and powerful. Many of these people had characteristics with notable historical figures like Julius Caesar, and he realized it would be useful to collect these ideas into one book. In 1995, he shared his idea with Joost Elffers, a book packager.

The original version of what would become known as The 48 Rules of Power was released in 1998. The purpose of the book was to give readers the tools they need to either climb the ladder of power or fight back against people in positions of authority. Greene asserts that the book's 48 principles represent a synthesis of the wisdom of a wide range of historical figures, including Sun Tzu, Niccolò Machiavelli, Haile Selassie I, Queen Elizabeth I, Henry Kissinger, Carl von Clausewitz, P.T. Barnum, and numerous others.

Warren Buffett and Jay-Z are just two of the many famous people who have praised The 48 Laws of Power, declaring it a "paradigm mover," since its release. In fact, Jay-Z mentions the book in his rap verse for "PrimeTime," released in 2011.

The 48 Laws of Power has been a huge success, selling over 1.2 million copies in the US alone. Twenty-four further translations of the book exist. Fast Company termed the book a "massive cult classic," while the Los Angeles Times referred to Greene as a "cult here."

There has no doubt been a great deal of criticism leveled towards The 48 Laws of Power. Some have spoken out against the book, claiming it promotes immorality and a Machiavellian worldview. Others have referred to it as a "how to" guide for betrayers. Greene has said in reaction to these allegations, "Although critics may label these rules as "evil," successful business owners use them all the time. Truthfully, you're constantly on the lookout for methods to wipe out your competition, and this hunt can get pretty brutal."

Please note that this summary of The 48 Laws of Power by Robert Greene is NOT the original book. This book was written and published by Melody Jefferson and is not affliated with or endorsed by Robert Greene.

LAW 1:
DO NOT OUTSHINE THE MASTER

Always work to ensure that those in positions of control over you feel comfortable and confident in their superiority. It's not that you shouldn't make an attempt to impress or delight them, but going overboard could backfire. There is a possibility that you will cause them anxiety or insecurity.

You might be able to make them feel scared or unsafe.

Instead, you should work to make your "masters" appear more knowledgeable than they actually are if you want to rise through the ranks to power yourself.

LAW 2:
BE WARY OF FRIENDS AND LEARN TO USE YOUR ENEMIES

Be watchful of everyone, including your buddies. Since they are more likely to betray you than others, they are more inclined to feel envious of you. They are prone to developing a short temper and a spoilt attitude.

The people you know and trust should really inspire more fear in you than your enemies do. Seek for an old adversary if you need a dependable ally. This once-rival will be out for revenge. Look for ways to create enemies if you don't already have any.

LAW 3:
HIDE YOUR INTENTIONS

Don't explain your reasons for acting unless it's absolutely required. This keeps things very confusing. Having everyone else in the dark works to your advantage. Because they can't possibly defend themselves against you if they don't know why you're doing what you're doing.

The ability to deceive others purposely exists. Provide them with the false impression, surround them with smoke and confusion, and by the time they figure out your genuine motivations, it will be too late.

LAW 4:
SAY LESS THAN IS NECESSARY

Don't waste your time attempting to convince others with flowery language. Even if you are a linguist, the more you ramble on, the less impressive you will appear. It sounds like you're spiraling out of control and getting more desperate by the minute. Those with a smaller vocabulary seem more formidable. It's more likely that you'll say something careless the longer you chat.

There are circumstances where it would be inappropriate to remain silent. The absence of conversation raises questions. In these situations, you should always utilize ambiguous wording. If you are unsure about your situation, it will be tougher for others to deceive or defeat you.

LAW 5:
GUARD YOUR REPUTATION WITH YOUR LIFE

Reputation is the bedrock of authority. You can use intimidation to your advantage if you have the right kind of reputation. Yet if your reputation takes a turn for the worst, you open yourself up to attacks from every direction.

Know and control how other people perceive you. Pay attention to how you come across to others. Keep your outward appearance in line with how you want to be perceived and how you feel and think. Develop an unconquerable reputation. Monitor for any reputational attacks and intervene before they might cause damage.

Discover how to temporarily weaken your opponents by damaging their reputations. Then sit back and watch as public opinion destroys them.

LAW 6:
COURT ATTENTION AT ALL COST

The need for those who stand out from the crowd and rise beyond the norm is enormous. Hence, it's important to embrace opportunities to develop traits that set you apart and draw attention to yourself. Avoid avoiding controversy if doing so will benefit your reputation. It's better to be attacked than ignored, in almost all cases.

Everyone is judged based on first impressions. Putting it plainly, invisible things don't matter. If you fade into the background, you cease to exist. Stand out and be easily recognizable. Attract attention to yourself like a magnet. Put forward an inflated image of oneself by all means necessary. Do better and inspire those around you to do the same.

LAW 7:
HAVE OTHERS DO THE WORK, BUT ALWAYS TAKE THE CREDIT

All of humanity is like savage animals squabbling over scarce resources in a vast forest. Killing and hunting are ways of life for some. Some survive by preying on the unwary.

Never be afraid to take use of other people's help, knowledge, or expertise. In addition to saving you time and effort, this will also make you appear more efficient and as if you possessed skills and abilities that you did not. The focus should be on you, not your supporters. Time is a commodity that can't be replenished. Do not waste your time and effort. Don't waste your time doing something that someone else can do for you if you can find a way to put your own spin on it.

LAW 8:
MAKE OTHERS COME TO YOU

Aggressive people often lack self-control. Due to their limited vision, they are unable to consider the long-term repercussions of their aggressive behavior. Worse, their aggressive nature draws a wide array of opponents who are just as aggressive and, in some circumstances, more clever. When this happens, all of their aggression is diverted to somewhere else.

There is no use in competing if you feel like you have no control over the outcome and are instead forced to merely react. Action that is aggressive and action that is effective are two whole different things. It's wiser to stay back, consider your alternatives, and set traps for your opponent. Try to maintain your composure. Coerce others into taking action and coming to you, regardless of what they want. You'll feel powerful and in charge after you reach this goal.

LAW 9:
WIN ACTIONS, NOT THROUGH ARGUMENT

We're all well-aware of the power that language has to deceive. As words are slippery, arguments lack a firm foundation. Furthermore, even if we are persuaded to change our thoughts and agree with the arguer, we typically only need a short amount of time to revert back to our former viewpoint.

Even if we were to win an argument, the victory would be primarily symbolic. It's more likely that our opponent's fury will be powerful and long-lasting than any change in their opinion.

Using actions to influence people's beliefs is more powerful. Don't just explain it; demonstrate it.

LAW 10:
DON'T BE INFECTED BY THE UNHAPPY AND UNLUCKY

Like a contagious disease, an emotional condition can quickly spread to others. Stay away from negative people, as their sadness might spread to you and eventually kill you. If you try to make someone else feel better, you may believe you're helping, but in reality, you're just letting them bring you down with them. Instead, surround yourself with positive, successful individuals.

How do we know if we've found the infector? They're folks whose lives are always changing and who seem to have nothing but poor luck, broken relationships, and a general sense of discontent. You must quickly leave the area if you encounter such persons. Keep your distance and don't bother trying to be their pal. Let them alone and continue on. Don't try to argue with them. Don't bother asking anyone you know for assistance with them. Just avoid us if you possibly can.

LAW 11:
KEEP PEOPLE DEPENDENT ON YOU

In a world where things are scarce, those in most need take priority. If you want to be financially self-sufficient, you need to ensure that other people will constantly desire or need you. Dependability and trust in others is the key to independence. As long as other people rely on you, you have no reason to be afraid. If you are not necessary, however, you will be ignored as soon as feasible.

How can you make other people rely on you? Participate actively in the tasks assigned to you by your superiors and work hard to develop skills and expertise that are unique and indispensable (or, at least, the appearance of these talents and skills). Think forward to other possible sites or customers who may need your help.

LAW 12:
USE SELECTIVE HONESTY AND GENEROSITY TO NEUTRALIZE YOUR ENEMIES

Don't be afraid to treat everyone, even your enemies, with respect and honesty. The most vigilant of your opponents may let their guard down and forget about your less altruistic acts if you perform enough of them. You have a better chance of persuading and beating them when they are relaxed and vulnerable.

LAW 13:
APPEAL TO OTHER'S SELF-INTEREST, NOT THEIR MERCY OR GRATITUDE

We all need help from others at some point in our life. When you really need help from another person, don't try to make them feel sorry for you or bring up all the times you've helped them before. If you use these tactics, the other person will feel manipulated and will be less willing to help you.

Instead, focus on how your desired outcome from the interaction (or the relationship) can benefit the other person. Include that benefit in your sales presentation. Getting people to support you requires convincing them of the benefits they will reap from doing so.

LAW 14:
ACT LIKE A FRIEND, WORK LIKE A SPY

Possessing in-depth understanding about one's adversaries is essential for success. Make use of spies and play the role of a spy yourself to get as much data as possible. This will ensure that you are constantly one step ahead of the competition. You need to be able to ask relevant questions in order to function in society. Figure out where you stack up against the competition.

Do this consistently; don't stop doing it when you've achieved your goal. One never knows when such information can come in handy.

LAW 15:
COMPLETELY CRUSH YOUR ENEMY

It is essential to wipe out any potentially harmful adversary. Don't only render him helpless or weak. Keep going until you've killed him. If you don't wipe him down completely, he'll get back up and be an even more dangerous foe hellbent on revenge. Proceed until the task is completed. Destroy everything (in every sense of the word).

LAW 16:
ABSENCE INCREASES RESPECT AND HONOR

In the early stages of getting to know a new friend, partner, or business colleague, it's crucial to spend as much time as possible with them. You might as well give up on it if you don't make the beginning. If you've built a solid rapport with someone, it's not your presence but your absence that will make you truly shine.

You may have noticed that the more the pursuing partner in a long-term romantic relationship pursues the other, the less interest the pursued partner shows in the pursuing partner. Being too close to the pursuer can be dangerous. The pursued individual feels trapped since their ability to dream and imagine is being stifled.

The value of a commodity declines when there is an abundance of it. Making yourself easily approachable lowers your perceived value. After establishing one's reputation, it often helps to take a break.

One effective strategy is to exploit the perceived lack of availability. Items that are scarce are automatically held in higher favor. Common things don't warrant serious consideration, in my view.

LAW 17:
BE OCCASIONALLY UNPREDICTABLE TO KEEP OTHERS IN SUSPENDED TERROR

We're all creatures of habit that look for consistency and order in the world around us. Having people view you as predictable gives them a sense of power over you. People are continually analyzing your actions to determine your motivations. They will attempt to exploit your perceived uncertainty.

You can fight back against this by periodically resorting to a sneak assault. Keep the impossible completely out of it. This will make them defensive all the time, which will make them feel unsafe and untrusting of you. The more people try to make sense of what you're doing, the more confused they'll become.

LAW 18:
NEVER BUILD FORTRESSES TO PROTECT YOURSELF

The military views the construction of a castle for the sake of seclusion as a questionable strategy. As a result, you have no one to rely on but yourself, making you a sitting duck for your adversaries.

In a community, individuals can reach their full potential. Without social interactions and dependencies, humans would perish. Furthermore, while a fortress may appear to be the finest security against the dangers of the outside world, being isolated from the rest of society puts us in greater danger. We are a stationary, easy target and cut off from critical information and resources as a result of this. Avoid isolating yourself by living in a tower and instead spend time interacting with others. Gather support. Participate in ever-expanding social networks. To stay safe, take refuge in the company of others.

LAW 19:
UNDERSTAND WHO YOU'RE DEALING WITH, AND DON'T OFFEND THE WRONG PERSON

There is a wide variety of people in our globe. No matter how savvy you are, you can never predict with certainty how other people will react to you and your actions. If you make the wrong person feel bad, they might always hold it against you.

Hence, be wary of who you let to become your enemies and rivals. Don't fire your gun and hurt someone unintentionally. If you're going to do something that you know will offend someone else, at least try to be nice about it. It's never a good idea to make fun of someone, no matter how insignificant they may seem.

LAW 20:
DO NOT COMMIT TO OTHERS

Be on the outside of other people's fights if you don't want to get dragged into their drama. Be mindful of your allies and do all you can to assist them, but avoid taking a stance too quickly. You shouldn't take a stand on any one issue or side. Don't be afraid to turn people against one another in order to keep your freedom. Find a safe distance away from the fighting and observe what's going on. Wait before taking any action. The weary competitors will be easy to convince and defeat.

When you take a stance, everyone feels like they have control over you. Your former imposing demeanor has faded. If you don't take a stand, though, people will work hard to win you over. Let them expect your commitment but never feel it.

LAW 21:
PLAY DUMBER THAN YOUR MARK

One's intelligence level is a major factor in how others view them. Everyone enjoys thinking they're wiser than everyone else. That's why it's vital to never, ever, ever, ever, ever, ever, ever, ever, ever, ever, ever, ever, ever, ever, ever, ever, ever, ever, ever You need to make them feel like a genius. Indeed, you should elevate their sense of superiority above your own. Don't be afraid of making a fool of yourself. They won't be able to maintain their skepticism if you do this to them. Because you make people feel good about themselves, they will want to keep you around. And the more time you spend with them, the more subtlety you can exert your effect.

LAW 22:
USE SURRENDER TO TURN WEAKNESS INTO POWER

We all have our weak moments from time to time. That's great, so long as you have a plan for handling the situation. There's little point in fighting back if you're already in a weak position. Just give up and accept it. When your opponent concedes, you gain valuable time to gather your thoughts and wait for them to weaken. If you try to fight back, you'll probably end up losing. Hold off on taking back control until the time is right.

LAW 23:
CONCENTRATE YOUR FORCES

Finding a rich mine and digging it deeper and deeper is more lucrative than jumping from one shallow mine to another. Because of this, you should focus your energy where it will have the most significance. Focus on just a few things and give them your full attention. Securing essential resources and allies is crucial if you want to keep your influence and power over the long term.

LAW 24:
PLAY THE PERFECT COURTIER

Those with the most political clout and influence have control over everything in the globe. A talented courtier would thrive in this setting. What are some best practices for playing the role of a courtier? One who can strategically flatter superiors, behave respectfully in the face of peers, and wield dominance over subordinates in a subtle and graceful manner is characterized.

LAW 25:
RE-CREATE YOURSELF

You will feel the strain to fulfill a variety of roles that others have come to anticipate of you. Don't take either side, no matter how tempting. Construct a new identity that more accurately represents who you really are. Make something that will interest them without being tedious. Don't let other people define who you are; instead, take charge of the narrative that's being told about you. Keep up a public persona that is congruent with who you really are.

Those who are totally forthright should be avoided. Daily displays of emotion are appealing, but they might backfire if you come out as annoying or ashamed. Even if they manage to garner some initial support, in the long run their actions will only make them look weak and self-absorbed.

LAW 26:
KEEP YOUR HANDS CLEAN

Keeping your professional reputation in good standing is crucial to your career, and this depends less on what people see and more on what you decide to keep under wraps. Don't let your blunders or poor behavior bring shame on you. Maintaining an air of competence, authority, and refinement is essential at all times. You must always present the best possible image. Since we're all fallible, it's only human to try to cover up the fact that you messed up. Find something or someone to blame, and try to avoid dealing with the issue at hand.

In a same vein, avoid taking part in any immoral pursuits. The cat lends the monkey its paw in the fable "The Cat's Pay" so that the monkey might retrieve some chestnuts from the fireplace. In this manner, he can safely consume the chestnuts. Don't make oneself slog through an unpleasant task. If the task is too dangerous or disagreeable, look for someone else to take it on. Allow someone else to play the bad guy or deliver the terrible news.

LAW 27:
TAKE ADVANTAGE OF PEOPLE'S NEED TO BELIEVE

If you wish to exert influence, you need to amass a group of people who will do what you say they will. You may assume it's a major undertaking to build up this kind of fan base, but it's actually rather easy.

Seems all humans share a fundamental need to believe in something. Make yourself or your case the focal point if you choose. Give them more than simply something to believe in; give them a solid justification for their belief. Don't give any concrete promises or explanations. Don't rely on your rational mind, but on what you feel instead. Give your followers sacrifices and rites to perform in your honor. You will find that they are eager to lend a hand, and before long you will have a whole army at your disposal.

LAW 28:
ACT WITH BOLDNESS, NOT TIMIDITY

In general, people are rather shy. The natural inclination of the human race is to avoid dangerous situations. The goal of most people, at least in social situations, is to have a wide circle of friends and admirers. While we may all daydream of making a major life change from time to time, very few of us ever truly make the leap. It's because we're scared of the repercussions or of what other people may think. We prefer not to cause trouble or make ourselves an easy target.

Even if we try to justify our behavior as "practicality" or "care for others," it is still timidity. The lack of courage is a selfish trait. It's a manner of life in which one is preoccupied with one's own ego and the opinions of others.

Courage centers on helping others. It is the courageous who will go on to do what is great, not the timid. You should be brave and take action when you have strong feelings about something. That doesn't mean you should rush into something you haven't fully considered. As a result, this will have no bearing on the final outcome of your sentence. Instead, take a risk for a cause you care about.

LAW 29:
PLAN UNTIL YOU REACH THE END

Most people are confident in their abilities as futurists and planners. The public at large, however, is wrong. They make plans for the future based on what they believe will happen, but in actuality they are just giving in to their wants right now. They let their feelings lead them rather than their intellect. They abandon even the most comprehensive plans as soon as they encounter obstacles. Since they are preoccupied with their present feelings, they can't think ahead.

It's time to stop. Create a plan immediately and stick with it until the finish. And make sure you follow through on them. Be as detailed as possible in your planning. Consider both the worst-case and best-case scenarios. With this knowledge in hand, you will be less likely to be taken off guard in the future.

LAW 30:

MAKE YOUR ACCOMPLISHMENTS SEEM EFFORTLESS

Invest the time and energy necessary to research your topic, improve your abilities, and plan for the future, but make it seem as though your job was effortless. Don't brag about how smart you are or how much you pushed yourself. Don't bother pretending like you're making an effort. If your foes learn your plans and procedures, they can use that information against you.

LAW 31:

MAKE OTHERS PLAY WITH THE CARDS YOU DEAL

The most effective method of gaining someone's attention and sway is to give them a sense of mastery over a situation. When interacting with other individuals, it's helpful to present a range of solutions that would all result in the desired goal. Force them to choose between two alternatives, one of which is better for you but both of which is still bad. They think they have agency, but in reality you control every move they make.

LAW 32:
PLAY TO OTHERS' FANTASIES

We all have a natural inclination to run away from the truth when it's unpalatable or unkind. Don't bring up a sensitive subject in discussion unless you're ready to deal with the fallout. No one likes to face the fact that their problems more often than not stem from their own lack of skill and poor judgment. They prefer to place blame on others than take responsibility for their own problems.

Keep in mind that most people would rather live in a pleasant fantasy world than face unpleasant truths. We all do this, not just the mentally ill. Gaining access to those fantasies can give you a lot of strength. If you can make yourself a source of pleasure or comfort for those around you, you will gain power over them. Guarantee them the stars. Inspire them to create a fantastical self-portrait.

LAW 33:
DISCOVER OTHERS' WEAKNESSES

One of the most crucial skills is the capacity to identify and exploit other people's vulnerabilities, the weak spots in their psychological barriers. This frailty typically takes the form of a deep insecurity, a secret pleasure, or a powerful emotion or desire. You can put it to good use once you know what it is.

Of course, there are instances when words are easier to use than actions. Some people try to cover up their defects, while others proudly display them for all to see. So, how do we investigate these defects?

Pay close attention to people and what they say. Constantly put forth an attitude of empathy and genuine curiosity to break down barriers and encourage communication. If you let someone in on a secret, whether it's real or not, they may be more inclined to keep one of their own. Observe their faces and gestures in different settings. Find out who they look up to and who they despise.

LAW 34:
IF YOU WANT TO BE TREATED LIKE A KING, ACT LIKE ONE

To show their subjects or subordinates that they are approachable or have something in common with them, powerful people are sometimes tempted to adopt an air of the ordinary man. There was a blunder there. Because of this, they come to be looked down upon by society at large. As a result, there will be an undeniable erosion of public support for the leader, culminating in outright hatred.

If you want people to take you seriously, you have to carry yourself like a king. Kings have the utmost regard for themselves and expect (and usually receive) the same respect from their subjects. Performing with confidence and grace will make you feel like royalty.

LAW 35:
MASTER THE ART OF TIMING

The illusion of time is created through artificial means. Humans conceptualized the idea so that the infinite expanse of space may be simplified. Time may be altered and changed in numerous ways because it is a human construct. Time management is an essential ability. Never make it seem like you're in a rush, as this will make you appear unpredictable. Show an endless amount of patience, as if you already have everything you want.

Consider how the timing of your choices and actions can affect the outcome. You must learn to wait for the appropriate moment to act and then to seize it with both hands.

LAW 36:
IGNORING WHAT YOU CANNOT HAVE IS THE BEST REVENGE

It's just the way life is; sometimes you win, sometimes you lose. We have a habit of having the most difficulty obtaining our deepest desires. When we really want something, we work harder to get it. Ultimately, we cave to our cravings and serve them. As a result, we start to look very sad. When we let ourselves become paralyzed by anxiety over a problem or an aim, we fail to see the many strengths we already possess.

Nothing of the sort can ever happen. Instead than dwelling on what we can't have, we should push those desires away. We must demonstrate our complete and utter scorn for such ideals. This will only serve to downplay the gravity of the situation and give our enemies a false sense of security. When we can make the things we lack or that worry us seem unimportant, we gain a sense of control over them and our lives.

LAW 37:
CREATE COMPELLING SPECTACLES

In order to influence someone, it's best to appeal to their emotions. Some people simply cannot be convinced by arguments, evidence, or logic. Instead, people are affected deeply by vivid visuals and impressive symbolic actions. If you can convince someone to feel this way, you can get them to do practically whatever you want them to, or at the very least, forget that you're trying to control them.

LAW 38:
THINK WHATEVER YOU WANT, BUT BEHAVE LIKE OTHERS

It's possible that your way of thinking is unique. Don't let it show.

If you challenge the current quo, people will think you're trying to draw attention to yourself. They will perceive you as arrogant and dismissive of their needs. They will take what you do as a personal attack on their culture. They'll go to extremes to make fun of you if you dare to be unique.

Don't try to seem like a person who values other people's traditions and customs. Meet the locals and emphasize the ways in which you're similar to their culture. Make sure you're just hanging out with like-minded people who won't raise an eyebrow at anything you say.

LAW 39:
TO CATCH MORE FISH, STIR UP THE WATERS

While the waves are calm, the enemy can plan their next move with greater ease. You need to construct a scene to attract the fish to the surface, where they may be caught more easily. If you can keep your calm under pressure, you can make your opponents more irrational.

Trouble can be caused most effectively by playing on the opponents' basest emotions, such as pride, rage, love, or vanity. The more angry they get, the more they'll completely lose it. Due to their disorganization, they are easy to defeat.

LAW 40:
DESPISE THE FREE LUNCH

Do not put your hope on giveaways. It's normal practice for deals to include hidden clauses that serve a greater purpose. If you want something badly enough, you should be willing to pay for it. In addition, when you pay for things on your own, you never have to worry about being in debt to anyone.

LAW 41:
AVOID STEPPING INTO A GREAT MAN'S SHOES

Something's original occurrence is always more remarkable and unique than subsequent ones. It's not enough to merely try to replicate the achievements of a great superior, father, sibling, or colleague who has come before you. If possible, double their rate of improvement.

To outshine them, use all the tools at your disposal. Don't wallow in their misery or fall into the same rut they have. Make your own way to the top and become a household name. Turn around when you need to. Go your own path and make an impression.

LAW 42:
TAKE DOWN THE SHEPHERD AND THE SHEEP WILL SCATTER

The common perception is that one troublemaker is to blame for a series of misfortunes. Often, there is only one person who is out to spread discord and turn the group against you. If you let them keep doing what they're doing, they'll attract even more followers. As soon as possible, make them harmless. Don't give them another chance to cause trouble, and avoid engaging in dialogue with them in the hopes of reaching a settlement. Take away their credibility and make them look like fools by isolating them from their followers. When the root of an issue is fixed, the problem goes away.

LAW 43:
WORK ON THE HEARTS AND MINDS OF OTHERS

Avoid coercion if you want other people to do what you want them to. While this may produce some short-term success, it almost always ends badly. Forcing something on someone makes them resent it and may lead to rebellion or plotting against you.

Instead of trying to force someone to do what you want, try to win them over with your charm. Make them eager to comply with your orders. Most easily seduced individuals are reliable team players.

You need to be able to articulate the way you make other people feel in order to master the art of seduction. Discover their weak spots and exploit them. Making an emotional connection with them can help you overcome their resistance. Use their worries and principles as negotiating tools. Think on the mental and emotional states of the people around you.

LAW 44:
USE THE MIRROR EFFECT TO DISARM

It's a surefire way to weaken your opponents if you imitate their strategies. If you want to fool them, you have to do what they say exactly. They will feel humiliated, ashamed, and furious, and as a result, they may lose their temper and explode. On the other hand, it may convince them that you are a leader who shares their values and ideas.

LAW 45:
PREACH THE NEED FOR CHANGE, BUT MAKE CHANGE GRADUAL

The fact that we all know novelty may be good doesn't stop us from being creatures of habit. People might become upset and even rebel when forced to deal with too much change, any change.

If you're just getting started or in a position of power, it's best not to try to make enormous, sweeping changes all at once. Instead, take small, manageable steps while demonstrating a healthy respect for the existing quo. Make the modifications as unobtrusive as possible.

LAW 46:
DO NOT APPEAR TO BE TOO PERFECT

It's perilous to try to make oneself look better than other people, and it's even riskier to try to make yourself look like you have no flaws. Being the target of others' jealousy increases the likelihood of harm being attempted against you.

It's necessary to occasionally showcase those shortcomings if you don't want to come across as too perfect. Accept your tiny shortcomings and use them to your advantage. If you do this, people will perceive you as more sociable and less envious.

LAW 47:
IN VICTORY, LEARN WHEN TO STOP

Don't let your guard down or get too carried away with jubilation. Even if you win, you can find yourself severely defenseless soon after. When you're feeling confident and bold after a triumph, you're more likely to develop enemies.

Don't let your accomplishments make you cocky. Never stop pondering and plotting. When you've fulfilled your mission, it's time to call it a day.

LAW 48:
BE FORMLESS

Adopting a recognizable shape and announcing your goals leaves you vulnerable to attack. Instead of adopting a fixed form, stick to being formless and pliable. That is to say, keep moving. Remember that there is always an element of uncertainty and that nothing lasts forever. Keep your formless, liquid-like state as a shield.

Milton Keynes UK
Ingram Content Group UK Ltd.
UKHW010722200923
429044UK00001B/99